one carers tales

I Cared

The. Unseen. Carer

I Cared: one carers tales
First published in Great Britain in 2025
by: DAISA PUBLISHING
An imprint of PARTNERSHIP PUBLISHING

Written By The. Unseen. Carer

The editors have ensured a true reflection of the author's tone and voice has remained present throughout.

A CIP catalogue record for this book is available from the British Library.
ISBN 978-1-915200-92-1

Book Cover Design by: Partnership Publishing
Book Type Set by: Partnership Publishing

Book Published by:
PARTNERSHIP PUBLISHING
Lincolnshire, United Kingdom
www.partnershippublishing.co.uk
Printed and bound by CPI Group (UK) Ltd, Croydon, CR0 4YY

Partnership Publishing is committed to a sustainable future for our business, our readers and our planet. This book is made from paper certified by the Forestry Stewardship Council (FSC), an organisation dedicated to promoting responsible management of forest resources.

one carers tales

I Cared

The. Unseen. Carer

To family and friends, some sadly no longer around, to those who may have thought they were just doing their job and to random strangers who made my life easier:

To JJ, without whose help this time would have been a lot harder, and to T, uncomplaining reader and critical friend of my scribblings.

Contents

Introduction

The second Thursday in December that year wasn't a normal day but I had enjoyed a similar Thursday in several Decembers past.

The evening before, I met my parents at a Carol Concert on my way home. I was always just in time for this, once arriving as the organisers had stopped taking money and it was about to start!

At the literary lunch on the Thursday three authors entertained us after a good meal. My parents attended five or six of these each year and invited me to the Christmas one. The authors in February sounded interesting, though, and I said so.

"We'll go as long as I'm not having my operation" – first I knew of it – I was told. I hoped they wouldn't clash.

Even then, a little overshadowed, that Thursday didn't seem like the end of an era.

Operation and luncheon clashed but the "patient" wanted me to go to the February lunch. Alone, it turned out, when some friends also dropped out. To decline would have been to show how worried I was.

The operation was the day before. Parent was, I gathered that morning, out of intensive care. So I went. There was drama later that day, but after a few days parent returned home.

Home, but health not fully restored. There would be a couple of falls that year. Parents went to their last lunch in March. We wouldn't go to that concert or meal, usually as then on successive days, together again.

Just over a year later my annus horribilis started. The other parent was taken ill suddenly and died after three difficult months. Surviving parent deteriorated. I became redundant.

I looked for work for a while at a difficult time then decided to look after surviving parent who could not remain at home otherwise.

I attended to their physical needs and financial affairs – "cared" in every sense of the word. Somewhere, dementia crept in.

I don't regret my choice. I saw some of the best of human kindness and customer service (and a few poor examples of the latter too).

Those December Thursdays will sadly never return but now I yearn for a new normal, sharing my skills - professional, literary, experience gained from looking after an elderly person or the foreign languages I have had too few opportunities to use - and contributing again to society.

...

I wrote some short pieces for myself about the experience of caring at the time. Therapy probably.

The incidents described happened. I and occasional contributor Boris (not *that* one) have used fictional names for the few companies which earned the Fawlty Towers Memorial Prize for Customer Service. No doubt they have improved considerably since we dispensed with their services and our purpose is to illustrate best practice, not name and shame. As stated above there are many more bouquets than brickbats to award.

When were the pieces written? Over a period of time and in the order in which they appear. Some contemporary references will give readers a clue but it doesn't matter. The messages are timeless.

So here are my Carer's Tales.

I have called myself "The Unseen Carer" because that is what it often felt like.

These are "One Carer's Tales" because every carer will have different experiences though our rollercoasters will certainly be emotional and probably physical mental and financial too.

You may call me Olav Persson if you wish. It isn't my name but it means something to me.

Gotcha?

...

“I was innocently walking through the flower bed when a bird suddenly dropped down from the sky next to me. It was obviously dead. I was quite shocked and thought I would pause a moment and pay my respects, like.”

OR:

“It’s a fair cop, Guv.”

Cats do not, as far as I know, speak English (though in that well known feline documentary “Top Cat” they speak American. They also appear in a wider variety of colours than I have seen).

I grew up with two of them and they can communicate effectively, certainly on matters of importance to them, though I never attempted to hold a conversation during which a Solicitor ought to be present....

If I had been able to speak to the neighbour’s cat on that day shortly after I began to look after Pat, I would most likely have received the first answer. Whether I would have believed it is a different matter....

Pat is, like me, a cat person, but not at the expense of birds to which they might pose a threat.

Investigating the circumstances of the bird's death was not practical but I had an idea which might prevent such things happening in our garden in the future.

Many years ago we had a wooden bird table, hand crafted by a friend of a Great Aunt, which sadly rotted and was eventually discarded. It had never been replaced. Now was the time to do so. The new one would be metal and readily available, purchased from a local pet supplies business, not the lovingly crafted item I remember from childhood days. I am not practical and I don't know anybody who could recreate such a beautiful thing.

Buying a new bird table, which can be seen from the dining room window, was a good move. I am happy to report that there has been no recurrence of the incident in the garden.

We do not blame cats for their natural instincts. I have fond memories of watching our black and white cat from childhood days, who clearly fancied himself as the world's greatest hunter, engaging in a well worn routine on our lawn. Just as he was poised to strike, the birds would have other ideas, such as flying off. It was hilarious.....

He "succeeded" only once. On that occasion my Mother managed to rescue the bird from him, though not without some difficulty. He was evidently proud of himself and very reluctant to let go of his prey.

Sadly my Mother was called upon to – and did – rescue rather more birds from the jaws of his grumpy Mother. (He was an "accident", coinciding with his Mother's first Birthday, but certainly well loved by us if not her. The interaction of their two different characters was at times very entertaining). She was small and slender while he was large and at times clumsy. She was sometimes assertive, to be polite; he, timid.

She stood out much less than he did – doubtless enabling an aerial warning system to operate in his case - and I suspect he also created mini earthquakes as he walked across the lawn.

Making the garden much safer for birds is reason enough to justify the purchase of the bird table but it is not the only one. A variety of birds, small and large, use it and other regular visitors include squirrels, who sometimes engage in all sorts of acrobatics to get nuts out of the holder. Having shown off their skills they often proceed to bury the nuts somewhere in the lawn. Watching all this has given Pat and me much pleasure over the years. Above all, though, for Pat, who rarely goes out, it has been good to bring that interest home.

So I will reserve judgement on the neighbour's cat and the incident which caused me to buy the bird table in the first place……

A Quarter of a Century of Carers Tales

Contents

one carers tales no.1

How It All Began

...

My name is not Olav Persson, though that *nom de plume* might help a handful of people who know me well to guess who I am. The person I look after is entitled to their privacy and so – as a carer – am I.

Let me tell you something about myself, however. Five years ago I was approaching my fiftieth birthday and working as a professional. My parents were in good health for their ages and lived their lives independently.

Was my life carefree? Not at all. My job gave me a lot of stress, one parent had been ill the previous year and the other was facing an operation, which we trusted would be routine. So far, so fairly typical for somebody of my age, you might think.

So why do I look back on those days now as days of innocence? Undoubtedly because of what has happened since.

During an *annus horribilis* a couple of years or so ago, I lost one parent, saw the speedy decline in health of the other to the point where they were no longer able to function independently and then lost that job.

Each of those events was painful in its own right. I was

determined at least to return to work as soon as possible and set out to do so against a difficult background.

My efforts did not bear fruit but after a short period of time I came to a realisation. The needs of my surviving parent – let us call that person Pat – gave me two choices. I could either put Pat in a nursing home and make every effort to get back into employment or become a full-time carer.

Let me make something absolutely clear. There have been some well-publicised exceptions, but I believe that nursing homes do a very valuable job. Their staff are almost certainly undervalued by society for looking after those who are dearest to us. They are generally very kind people.

Pat has, like many older people who live in their own homes, spent some time in a nursing home. My comments about them are based on real experience, not general impressions.

Pat has coped with being in a nursing home, for six weeks or more on one occasion, better than I would have expected. This has always been on the basis that it was a temporary measure and Pat would return home when "they" allowed it. There have perhaps been times when, if I had been Pinocchio, my nose would have grown a little longer.

I have never been sure how Pat would cope with the prospect of not returning home. We never discussed care during the good times and we are not able to do so now.

So I opted to become a full-time carer. Looking back on my life five years ago, its normality seems like bliss to me. I would love once more to be among those who travel to work in the morning and return home in the evening. Their responsibilities are defined by the working day, even though I know that many also take work home with them, physically or mentally, as I did. So I know I am wearing rose-tinted specs here, but it doesn't stop my nostalgia....

Twenty-four hour care of a person means just that: helping them to bed in the evening and to get up in the morning, attending to their needs if they wake up during the night or can't sleep. I do a considerable amount of paperwork on Pat's behalf and have attended meetings without number with professionals interested in the welfare of older people. Various carers perform specific tasks during the day or sit with Pat when family are not there - one is doing so while I write this - but such carers need to be organised and paid.

Society probably sees me either as a full-time carer or as unemployed (though I have never held myself out to anybody as being so). I could reply to the latter judgement that I have never not worked so hard in my life, but I prefer to think of myself as more than a label. Being a carer is hard work and considerably restricts my freedom. It can be interesting, fulfilling and occasionally funny too. It has taken me a long way out of my comfort zone.

If I had known then what I know now....but I do it because Pat is worth it, to paraphrase the TV advert. I want society to understand a little more about the life of carers, for I fear that their experience is very much hidden.

one carers tales no.2

Upon Quaint Ceremonies...

...

At the State Opening of Parliament, when Black Rod* is about to summon Members of the House of Commons to go to "the Other Place" (as MP s evidently call the House of Lords) to listen to the Queen's Speech, the door is famously slammed in his face. He then knocks three times on the door, is admitted, summons the MP s and in due course everybody trundles to the Lords' Chamber. Job done, with the benefit of rather colourful ceremony.

BR (as I'm sure his friends don't call him) would be disconcerted if the response to his knocking was a cry of: "Go away, Rodders. It doesn't matter how many times you bang your mace. We're not letting you in!" He would be equally surprised if the response was: "Don't stand on ceremony, Rodders. Do come in. Let's not bother with all that slamming of doors business – it's rather old hat."

Incidentally, the purpose of this ceremony is to show that Members of Parliament are not subservient to the Crown.

You may be wondering why, as a carer, I was reminded of that quaint old ceremony. Let me explain....

Pat is looked after by a particular carer, Gerda, for about fifteen hours a week. Before Gerda was appointed, it was suggested to us that a specific care account should be set up, to receive the contributions from both Pat and the Local Authority and out of which the carer would be paid.

Pat set up such an account with a "Friendly Society" recommended by Social Services. The carer records her hours on a timesheet each week and this, duly countersigned by me, is posted to the "Payroll People" every four weeks. A weekly standing order is paid into the care account, to avoid large amounts going out of Pat's account every four weeks.

At the end of the first four week period, I checked that the account held sufficient funds to pay Gerda as well as the fees of the "Payroll People". I rang and Pat authorised the people at the Friendly Society to give me the relevant information. I soon discovered that I would need to telephone each time Gerda's hours were submitted, as calculating the balance of the Friendly Society account in my head was as easy as working out the scores of the contestants in "QI" before Stephen Fry announces them. (I hasten to add that I am not a Professor of Mathematics).

On one occasion when I rang, a young lady told me that they could not give this information. I pointed out that they had authority from Pat to do so.

"Oh, I know", she replied, "but we've changed our system."

Whilst I could be thankful the account had not been opened with an Unfriendly Society, this was – to say the least – rather inconvenient. At my request, the young lady then put me through to a colleague who gave me the relevant information without further ado.

The second time the young woman said this, I was once again somewhat alarmed by her words, but after I had gone through this little ceremony several times I became used to it. Was the young woman, I wondered, related to Black Rod? If so, maybe she relished the opportunity of (metaphorically, obviously) slamming the door in somebody else's face? Perhaps her name was Roderica Black?

Be that as it may, sometime later the "Payroll People" suggested that it would be more convenient if Pat opened an account with their bank (which happened to be Pat's also). So Pat did. I would like to say that everything has worked like clockwork since. I would also like to say that I won several millions on the lottery last week. I am told, by people who know more about the latter subject than I do, that you have to buy a ticket first.

I have a confession to make, though. I feel a certain nostalgia for those telephone calls when I was told that the system had changed. If Roderica had simply given me the information immediately, life would have been so much duller. If on the other hand her colleague had repeated the line about system changes, my blood pressure would have sky-rocketed. As it was, it was a harmless and rather quaint ceremony, even if I'm not quite sure what it symbolised....

Roderica, if you're reading this, I miss you. Life is rather less colourful without you....

**At the time this piece was written, Black Rod was a man. In February 2018 Sarah Clarke was the first female to be appointed to that position. Her official title is Lady Usher of the Black Rod.*

one carers tales no.3

For Bob's a Jolly Good Fellow...

...

It was never difficult to decide what to give Pat as a Birthday or a Christmas present. I always bought a book. The only thing I had to think about was which one.....

For the past four years or so, Pat has not been able to read, the loss of a very great pleasure. So I had to choose a different gift. I am afraid that I have not used a great leap of imagination. I moved from books to chocolates.

A couple of years ago, a Waterstones e-mail alerted me to the publication of James Bowen's book "A Street Cat Named Bob". That dealt with the problem of what to buy for my brother and sister-in-law, but I had a childhood memory and a thought crossed my mind.

When I was twelve, my Mother was still reading to me towards the end of the day. It was not that I was unable to read myself – indeed, I would then read a different book for a while before "lights out". I have a very vivid memory of listening to "Watership Down" whilst we were on holiday in Scarborough when I was that age. My room was on the fourth floor of a sea-front hotel whilst Mum and Dad were staying (at least) two floors lower. I suspect that this tradition died out shortly afterwards.

Nevertheless, if I had enjoyed it when Mum had read to me, perhaps I could buy James Bowen's book and Pat would enjoy being read to? I decided to try it.

Pat has always loved animals. For those unfamiliar with "A Street Cat Named Bob", it is the story of a cat which "adopts" a Big Issue seller, gives him a purpose and enables him to tackle some deep-rooted problems in his life. I have always had the greatest respect for those selling the Big Issue – even more so after reading this book and its sequel – and it is a truly heart-warming story. This proved to be a great success, so I continued with the experiment. Pat has now listened to quite a few animal stories, including Susan Finden's delightful "Caspar the Commuting Cat".

I try to vary the reading to provide the greatest possible mental stimulation. Pat used to be interested in current affairs and would always express well-informed opinions.

A little over four years ago, we watched coverage of the election of a Labour Leader. While waiting for the result, I told Pat a story from Simon Hoggart's biography of Michael Foot. Thirty years earlier Labour MPs alone chose their Party Leader. Already knowing the result, leadership candidates Michael Foot and Denis Healey entered a room full of MPs waiting to hear it. Healey was grinning broadly while Foot looked as if he had suffered a great shock. Healey's former deputy in Cabinet placed a bet on him with "Commons Bookmaker" and Labour MP Ian Mikado. Hoggart called this "the easiest ten pounds Mikado ever made". Foot had won.

TV Coverage showed the Miliband Brothers entering the conference room where the result of the election was to be announced. David seemed very happy. Ed looked as if he had received bad news.

There are no bookmakers in this story but it was clear to me that David Miliband had won. First round results were given. He was ahead.

"I'm going to make a prediction," said the man from the Beeb, "that David Miliband has won."

"Oh, no, he hasn't" I thought as if the Beeb was presenting an interactive pantomime and with equal and opposite conviction to mine of just moments before. I had read in my boss's copy of *The Times* that he needed to be nine per cent ahead on the first round. He wasn't (and he didn't).

Some years before that, Pat had shown me Jonathan Aitken's book "Heroes and Contemporaries", and specifically the Chapter on Lord Longford. I had been doubly surprised: that Aitken should have written a chapter on a man so unlike him and that Pat should have appreciated this short biography. When I read it myself I could see why. Widely ridiculed by the press, Longford seems to have been a very genuine and selfless man most of whose work with prisoners was away from the public domain. Remembering this, I selected it as another book to read.

Almost all of the books I have read to Pat are new to me. Any swear words I edit out. (As an aside, at Christmas I read a story about a vet, which was generally charming and well-written but featured on one occasion the word which Kenneth Tynan infamously uttered on television for the first time in the 1960s. A question to the author and publishers: Why?).

I try to avoid unhappy endings or "gory details". Some animal books may be delightful but have sad endings. Mike Pannett's tales of life as a North Yorkshire Policeman – grittier than the excellent Constable books by Nicholas Rhea which formed the basis of the TV series Heartbeat – are well written but occasionally feature memories of incidents which I would not wish to read to an older person who is (virtually) housebound. In such cases, I sometimes omit whole sections or a Chapter – so the smooth narrative might grind to a slightly jerky halt before I decide where to pick up the story again.

I have most recently shared James Bowen's second book "The World According to Bob" (an interesting reminder, among other things, that not everything in a writer's life changes when their first book is published).

I generally read to Pat two or three evenings a week and both of us enjoy it. Seeing the advertisement for James Bowen's first book gave me the idea. Bob is indeed a Jolly Good Fellow – in more ways than he could imagine.....

one carers tales no.4

The Case of the Missing *Yorkshire Post* (and other Exciting Events)

Spoiler: This piece was *not* written for, and subsequently omitted from, the new collection of Miss Marple stories.

...

"Off you go!" Gerda, Pat's German carer, bade me before each of the two Grand Days Out mentioned here. I know that she did, because she always says that when she arrives.

I should mention, as it is relevant to both of these trips, that I completed writing what I regarded as the novel of the century almost three years ago.

I vividly remember, as a student more than thirty years ago, sitting in the Junior Common Room of my College reading (a College copy of) the Yorkshire Post. That newspaper was and remains a broadsheet. The front page was most unusual for its day: a picture of the Humber Bridge, then nearing the end of its construction, took up half of it. The centre section of the bridge was being put in place. Unfortunately, I did not go out and buy a copy of that newspaper, which would have saved much subsequent heartache. For I wished to use the date of it in my work of fiction: trust me, the date on which that picture was published was relevant to Chapter Four!

One thing I knew: I had seen that picture whilst I was a student, during termtime, in the academic year 1980/81. The fact that the Humber Bridge opened in the summer of 1981 confirmed the period of publication, as the photograph obviously pre-dated the opening.

When writing the story, I used a date, which I didn't think was plucked from thin air: 4th June 1981. I was fairly sure that I had seen the picture either in the second, or more probably third, term of that academic year. My first contact with the archive was by telephone. They told me that they could search the archive for me, but would charge to do so. However, they very kindly looked at the newspapers within a few days of that date – and drew a blank.

With an old friend from Primary School days, Gerry, I headed to Leeds to search through the (microfiche) archives. We looked through all the papers from the term time between October 1980 and June 1981. I found some fascinating stories as I tried to be disciplined and look at front pages only. The good news is that I could be thankful I had not asked the keepers of the archive to undertake this task for me: I would have run up a considerable bill. The bad news is that I also drew a blank. A different date and event would have to be used for Chapter Four instead!

The second day out was to lodge a copy of the manuscript with a potential publisher I had read about. The address was a Pennine village, accessible by rail. It was accessible by road, too, but I didn't want the hassle of having to park there – and I am quite fond of train journeys, so it was a good excuse. Once again, Gerry accompanied me.

Global HQ turned out to be a little terrace house with an elderly car parked outside. The fact that it was HQ was marked by a plaque in the window. I knocked on the door, looking forward (a little nervously) to meeting the CEO. I knocked several times. I fancied I heard movement in the house, but the door didn't open so I may have imagined it (or the CEO may have heard some lunatic knocking on his door and decided to make himself scarce). In any event, I pushed my large envelope through the somewhat awkward letter box.

I knew that this was not a day I would ever describe in soundbites. I could feel the Hand of History upon me....

Gerry and I then went and found somewhere to eat and had a particularly expensive lunch. It seemed appropriate to celebrate such an important day. The advance would more than cover the cost in due course.

Travelling back on the train, I wondered whether I might already have missed a telephone call about my magnum opus? If so, the man to whom I had given an opportunity to spot my literary genius would just have to be patient.

I need not have worried. Nobody called in the next week – or month – either. Four months after my second day out, regretting that I had not done so earlier, I e-mailed to find out what was happening. "Nothing" it seemed. My manuscript was identified when I pointed out that it was hand-delivered. My carefully selected publisher did not publish that sort of thing and it was returned in the stamped addressed envelope I had included with the original delivery.

I was four months older and wiser – but, perhaps surprisingly, I still look back on a Grand Day Out (or Two).

Update:
I long ago gave up the effort of looking for a publisher for my magnum opus. Reading it is probably the literary equivalent of eating three Weetabix for breakfast.

I originally called this piece "A Grand Day Out (or Two)".

one carers tales no.5

A "Mailstrom" on the Hall Carpet

...

About six years ago, I sent a cheque to a charity featured on the Sunday morning BBC Radio 4 Appeal. A while later, a Close Relative, sharing the same uncommon surname and who is sadly no longer with us (and whom I shall henceforth call CR), was surprised to receive a request from that charity to gift aid the donation recently received.

CR worked long hours as a professional for more than forty years and was one of the most generous people I have ever met. I don't know whether, in retirement, dealing with the post became a substitute for work. What I do know is that CR was plagued by a large amount of mail – up to twenty items a day.

CR felt an obsessive need to respond to this. On one occasion, this convinced Roveriste wrote to a Toyota dealership declining its kind invitation to the launching of a new model. In vain did I point out that the garage only wanted to know who would be there, not who would not.

So far, so amusing. Readers will appreciate that twenty items of post a day do not consist solely or mainly of utility bills or personal missives, although those were of course sometimes received. They were mainly begging letters from charities and junk mail – if those are separate categories. A very large proportion were sent from three UK depots, one apparently owned by a foreign (non-EU) national Post Office.

I found it very worrying that CR could be identified as the probable donor to a charity which I had supported. Somewhere, a list must be circulating of "the generous" - or "gullible" in their eyes - predominantly elderly, people who could be relied upon to give to charities they had not heard of or to be persuaded that they might have won monies in foreign lotteries that they hadn't actually bought tickets for.

I never ceased to be amazed at the imaginative, official sounding names of companies which advised of large sums of unclaimed monies, details of which they would impart to CR (and, obviously, others) upon payment of a modest fee, in case they should be entitled to a share. I can't be sure, but I don't believe my relative ever sent a cheque to these companies at their foreign PO box numbers.

I know that CR did send for overpriced sweets and quackery, advertised in letters whose envelopes bore words such as "You have won £8500". CR sent a lot of letters each day. Did the possibility of getting some return influence these purchases?

I don't know. To me, though, those words on the envelope were clear and could not be subject to any small print among the enclosures. They were either true – in which case cheques to CR must have been lost in the post on a regular basis – or untrue. As they seemed to be the latter, it frustrated me that my relative dealt with such people.

Some time ago, there was a debate on a political website about whether people on the electoral roll should continue to be able to remove their names from the list sold commercially. Some marketing companies considered that this limited their business opportunities. One contributor argued that they had nothing to hide and nobody should have a reason to conceal their details. The first part of their statement I do not doubt: as to the second, I wanted to scream at my computer. Many junk mailers conceal their identity, hiding behind a PO Box or frequently a "Postbus" which I guess is the Dutch equivalent. They also deliberately target elderly, vulnerable people.

On the subject of the electoral roll, I was infuriated by my local authority's insistence that voters needed to select that particular "opt-out" each year, as many voters will have assumed that if their details were otherwise correct, they did not need to amend them in any way. I raised the issue with a local councillor, who told me that the authority was following legal advice on the issue. Obviously, I do not wish the Council to break the law at the expense of its local tax payers – but the law, in this case, was clearly an ass.

Twenty items of post a day for my late relative a few years ago is now down almost to zero, after much effort on my part, though the occasional charity still decides to revive communication after being dormant for several years. A plea to reputable charities: please do not do this. It can cause great heartache. Please also avoid promotions or lotteries which in any way resemble, and therefore legitimise, those of the unscrupulous.

The Royal Mail is paid to deliver letters. There are occasions, I am tempted to think, when it should be paid not to do so....

Update:

Following recent legislation charities are now careful to check their supporters' contact preferences to an almost absurd extent. I have had to reassure those which I support that I am very happy to hear from them. My comments are certainly not intended as an attack on the many worthy charities which exist both nationally and locally.

One charity recently wrote to CR, on the basis of donations made many years ago, but I have seen no other such letters for a long time. They received a phone call I have made a few times over the years: advising that CR is no longer around and requesting that, if they have not been in touch recently, they do not cause possible upset to relatives by trying to revive contact.

My local authority no longer seems to require the opt-out referred to above each year following the introduction of individual voter registration.

Second Update:

Has there been a leak of this piece before the book was published?

Has the post, a service I value and whose hard-working employees I salute, adopted my detailed corporate plan for it as set out in the final paragraph of my original article (but not necessarily in the way I had in mind)?

I didn't imagine post-free days when I first wrote it….

one carers tales no.6

At Your Service?

...

I was irritated that the man's system did not recognise the first and fourth digits of my X-figure banking passcode one Monday morning. When he threatened to cancel the number, I begged him not to do so. He then told me that "the system" had cancelled the number which I always remembered by thinking of the word "Peugeot".

Rather than thinking of the economic value of financial services and the tax revenues they provide, I consoled myself that I would simply have to go through a longer ID process and give my great grandfather's favourite colour if I needed to use telephone banking again in the next few days.

The following Thursday, I did. It was nearing the end of Gerda's four-week pay period and I needed to transfer some monies to the Friendly Society care account by the following Monday. We were about to spend a long weekend away and I still had much packing to do.

The first person I spoke to said, in effect, no X-figure banking passcode, no transfer to third party bank account. I patiently explained that my lack of passcode was due to the Bank's error earlier in the week. The fact that regular transfers were made to this account also seemed immaterial. After a long quarter of an hour, I was put through to another operative. In the Internet Banking Section. I explained for the second time that I didn't have internet banking and no, I couldn't go to a Branch to sort this matter out. Further, it needed to be sorted that day. The person in the Internet Banking Section couldn't understand why I had been put through to her. She wasn't the only one.

The third conversation was on more familiar territory. It mirrored the first one. I lobbed in the fact that, if anybody suffered financial loss for the failure of the bank to carry out the requested transaction, I would, of course, look to the bank to provide recompense. Something I regretted not saying earlier.

Number Four was a manager. At one point in the conversation she said: "As far as I'm concerned, you must have given the wrong digits to the telephone service on Monday and I'm not going to discuss that matter any further."

I replied: "As far as I'm concerned, I gave the correct digits as requested to the man on Monday and I'm not going to discuss *that* any further."

We did not get married.

Ultimately, fifty-five minutes into the call, Number Four agreed to transfer the monies. She did so and then, in effect, added: "Don't do it again."

"Excuse me!" I thought to myself. "Shouldn't I have been saying that to the bank?" Surely, what the Bank could do in fifty-five minutes, they could have done in five, by putting me through to the right member of staff. A good example of very poor customer service.

My friend Boris (not *that* one) reports that he tried to arrange a GP home visit on a specific date for Hilary, whom he looks after, to review medicines. He was told that the technology (a notepad, as in a pen and paper) could do it. The Government didn't object to advance booking but the senior partner did. Could he book it on the day? Enough said.

There is a public house in the Dales where the landlady reminds me of a Chairman of the Magistrates' Bench dealing with a particularly recalcitant offender (me!). I hope she doesn't know who she is. Readers may assume that I cite this as another example of poor customer service. Not so.

Not only does that pub offer a fine dining experience, said landlady has been particularly attentive to Pat's needs over the past few years. We sit at a table near the entrance and she ensures that Pat has a cushion and is comfortable. We discovered that gem of a place some time ago when Pat was in good health and independently mobile. I am glad that, when we found it, we looked beyond the obvious. The landlady, whatever our first impressions, is good-hearted and well-supported by her team.

Still in the Dales, I commend the volunteers on the Wensleydale Railway who treat Pat like Royalty, thereby making a wonderful day out for all of us as we relax and enjoy the scenic ride on their line.

Planning days out is more difficult when dealing with people who are frail. Managing the affairs of another person is a heavy responsibility. I have learned to judge the quality of service based on how well people look after Pat when we are together. Those who cheerfully lighten the burden are worth their weight in gold. There are plenty of good examples out there....

one carers tales no.7

A Tale of Two Hotels

...

A while ago we booked a weekend at a Hotel on the coast at which we had previously stayed. Making the booking, I was made well aware that this Hotel was owned by a large company and run on stalinist lines from afar. Bookings were accepted for Monday to Friday and Friday to Sunday or Monday, presumably so that unsold rooms can be used by the coach parties which form a large part of its occupancy.

We needed a room with easy access to the lift for Pat. The Hotel could allocate such a room to us, but Head Office might undo their handywork. To ensure we actually got this room, we needed to pay an additional £X fee to the company. Quite why Head Office would interfere with our booking in this way I have never been sure, but we paid up. It was too late to book a guaranteed parking space. We would have to take our chance with others for a space in the main (unreserved) area of the car park – which meant we needed to arrive early on the Friday afternoon.

Upon arrival – I had intended to be there by One O' Clock and got there four minutes late – we went to reception, expecting to collect our keys. We hadn't read the small print.

Keys were available for collection from Three O' Clock, even though the rooms had already been serviced. We could leave our luggage in an unlocked room, if we so wished. We didn't.

Circumstances had changed since our booking. Sadly, Pat had been in hospital after a fall and was now in a nursing home to regain mobility. After careful thought, we had decided to go ahead with the stay. We had received a ten per cent refund in respect of Pat's cancellation. We were surprised to be seated at the back of the dining area, having previously alerted the hotel to Pat's limited mobility. (The dining room did not have wheelchair access but we did not at the time of booking need this). It was possible, but we thought unlikely, that the hotel had amended its seating plan following our very late cancellation of Pat's stay.

Let me be fair to Joseph Stalin Holidays Plc (not their real name). The rooms were good. Mine had a brilliant sea view (an extra but I did not begrudge it). The waiters at table, receptionists and other staff we dealt with were, almost without exception, first class. I gave them a very good write-up on their comment card on Sunday morning.

Sunday morning! I never handed that card in, but that was the least of my worries. Wishing to make best use of the time, I put my suitcase and some other items in the car before breakfast but left my (elderly) toilet bag in the bathroom, a carrier bag and (in clear view of anybody who opened the door) a book on the table. (Matthew Parris, since you ask). It was at least an hour and a half to checkout time and lots of people who were with coach parties were leaving.

When I returned to an empty room, I was so shocked I wondered if I had misread the number. I hadn't. I eventually found a cleaner who, after some explanation, produced a bin bag containing my toilet bag and somebody else's used fizzy drink can. Matthew Parris had fared a little better, having apparently been lodged at reception. A bookmark of some sentimental value had been written on.

Before leaving, I expressed concern about this. A very professional young receptionist took notes and made soothing noises before a senior colleague decided to take over. She said that, although items had been left in the room and it was well before checkout time, the clearing of rooms if there was no case or coat left in them was "Company Policy". Stalin Plc's reply to my letter, written only because the "Manager" inflamed the situation by defending the indefensible, echoed this. It also apologised. Everybody had followed "Company Policy" so I am not sure why it did so.

We have just stayed at another resort, not a million miles from the first, happily this time with Pat. The staff at the second hotel were also first class. They work for a small family owned concern. A request for cheese on toast, not on the breakfast menu, was not too much trouble and didn't require a call to HQ. We didn't get there before 3pm, but if we had I don't doubt the key would have been given to us if the room was ready. The staff did everything we could have asked of them and were brilliant with Pat.

If I was running Joseph Stalin Plc, I would ask my staff to use common sense and not follow silly rules. I would ensure that cleaners service rooms vacated by coach travellers and not those where guests have not yet checked out. Oh, and ask my Managers: When there's nothing to be said, why does some fool always say it?

one carers tales no.8

Good Morning, Employers

...

Politicians – generally those who are in power at any particular time – frequently express their wish to see people working rather than claiming out-of-work benefits. This message has much support in the media. As someone who, about twenty years ago, found myself looking for work for a little while, I completely agree. Nothing is more frustrating than wishing to earn your own living and contribute to society and being denied the opportunity to do so.

So I wish that those same politicians and the media would spread another message, too. That there are many people who are unemployed but who are not at heart the idle layabouts of caricature. Redundancy can strike anyone: from a plant closure by a big multi-national deciding it can build iconic vans more cheaply in Turkey than the UK to professional firms merging and in the process displacing many longstanding employees and, in some cases, partners. Even in a healthy economy, these are everyday stories.

I write this because I feel that an image is sometimes created that those who are not working are doing so from their own choice. If the rhetoric is that they are good-for-nothings, why would an employer offer them a job? Yet if society won't give the unemployed a chance in roles they could fill, how can we criticise them for the circumstances they find themselves in?

So I would ask those politicians and the media to refine their message. It is absolutely right that people should "stand on their own two feet" as far as they are able to do so. There are also many people not in the labour market, for whatever reason, who wish to use their talents and who have skills to offer potential employers and society. Politicians should acknowledge this and employers should be encouraged where appropriate to get such people back into permanent employment, perhaps with the assistance of short-term subsidies.

I am not currently looking for work (nor holding myself out to anybody as doing so), but some, who don't know me well, may presume that I am unemployed. I concluded a while ago that I could not look after Pat and meet the demands of an employer without risking letting down both.

Many of those caring for elderly relatives can expect to find themselves looking for employment at some time in the future. This is a worrying prospect for the carer: will they face prejudice from prospective employers because of the time they have spent "not working"?

I can only use my own circumstances as an example. Over and above my normal duties, I was a sole signatory to business cheques and bank transfers in my most recent position. In the absence of my boss who normally did this, I authorised one payment of a million pounds as well as many such payments of six-figure sums. I have also authorised payment of my own (and others') salaries – I'm not sure which is the more scary but both require considerable trust in the office cashier!

I have also gained many skills from being a carer, as well as making full use of those from my professional background. I am organising another person's life: dealing with many professionals concerned with Pat's welfare; ensuring that somebody is in the house twenty-four hours per day; Pat needs to be fed and take tablets but also to go out as often as possible and be mentally stimulated in every possible way. Pat is not able to pay bills and run finances. I, as the carer, have to do these things.

Pat is a relative. Carers look after relatives because they love them, but there is an emotional cost too. I regard each day as a working day, from getting Pat up first thing to putting Pat to bed at ten o' clock at night and hoping that my own sleep will not be disturbed unduly. Every day I make a list of jobs to be done over and above the routine caring activities. Yes, there are moments of relaxing and enjoying Pat's company each day, but such quality time is not typical. I wish it were otherwise. The carer's job is to organise and physically assist the person they are looking after.

That energy and loyalty might be available to a potential employer in the future, but only they will be able to accept or reject it. Perhaps the title of this piece should have read "Good Morning, Employers *and Politicians*." I hope that both might learn something from it.

Update:

The situation I imagined a few years ago when I wrote this is the one in which I find myself today. Perhaps I am now the Unseen Former Carer.

one carers tales no.9

Lions Led by...

...

During the last few years, while caring for Pat, I have been very aware of human kindness. This has been expressed in many small ways, from carers who care as well as doing the job to shopkeepers who still enquire after Pat, whom they have not seen for a long time. If we eat out, waiting staff usually make sure that Pat is comfortable and looked after before taking our order, while patrons stand aside and hold the door to let us in or out. We have experienced the same courtesy and kindness at tourist attractions and on heritage railways when we have been on holiday. Many of these are commercial transactions, but Pat brings out the best in people and I am grateful to all those who make our lives so much easier.

As a carer, I undertake many transactions on behalf of Pat. I am grateful when the people I am dealing with get things right, as they usually do, but irritated if they don't and I feel I am doing their jobs for them.

Planning ahead and knowing that somebody will look after Pat is important when I need to go out. So I was annoyed when, having rung an agency one Thursday morning to ask whether somebody could provide cover the following

Wednesday, I rang the following day to discover they couldn't, but were *writing* to me to tell me so. Despite the telephone conversation on the Friday morning, the letter was still sent out – under separate cover from a bill which was sent the same day. Both arrived on Monday, late as our post always is. The professional carer they usually send agreed that the back office was both incurring unnecessary expense and failing to provide timely information to me. A brilliant carer let down by failings in the back office.

Another company provides morning and occasional lunchtime calls to Pat. Towards the end of last year their service was interrupted during a period of recuperation in a nursing home. Looking at the first bill a few weeks after visits resumed, I thought immediately that there was an error in it. I recalled that visits had re-started on a Friday, not on a Monday as shown. My diary confirmed they had started the Friday *after* the date shown, though I would also have contacted the office if the error had been in our favour.

There were further errors in the bill (which was paid by Direct Debit) and Pat had been overcharged by about £100. I sent a detailed e-mail pointing out each incorrect entry. I received no apology but they disputed one visit, value approximately £6, where they said I had not given the required twenty-four hours notice of cancellation directly to the office. (I normally ring the office, even though the carers always promise to notify cancellations to them. On one particularly busy day, I relied on the promise. No carer called the following day but they wanted to charge).

I have two concerns about this. Most seriously, I am able to check Pat's bills and correct errors. I do not suspect dishonest intent, but similar errors on bills to many of their clients would not have been noticed and the company would have received monies they were not entitled to. If someone had discovered that at a later date.... Despite my helping them in this way, they chose to quibble about one visit they felt entitled to charge for. If I had charged the cost of my time in dealing with their errors and doing somebody else's job, my bill would probably have been more than that. I continue to use the company because of the quality of their front-line staff: I don't expect any of their employees to lose money, but the company should be willing at times to acknowledge its mistakes and pay for them. Another case of failings in the back office....

Something else which puts me in Grumpy Old Man mood. Pat's Doctor is excellent. We have sometimes wished to request visits when another relative is present, so that all of us know what the Doctor has to say. For this reason, we have wanted to arrange a visit for a particular date. The practice which looks after Pat has a policy that they will only arrange visits on the day, so that people either have to "ring at 8.30" or go to the surgery to request a visit. Neither options is necessarily practical for a full time carer, or others concerned with the care of an elderly person. (Incidentally, as I recall from times past, they are not particularly helpful to working people who have health concerns either).

I believe that such a practice arose because of targets, set in the late 1990s, relating to same-day visits by GP s. I recall Tony Blair squirming with embarrassment during a Leaders' Debate before the 2005 General Election, apparently blissfully unaware such a practice had arisen. I thought it had been completely discredited and have been surprised to meet it on a couple of occasions in the last year or so.

one carers tales no.10

Lend Me Your Ears...

...

What is a friend? Someone we need in our darker hours perhaps?

I have been blessed by many very good friends over the years, for which I am particularly grateful. Friends listen to us, we enjoy their company and at times they bear our burdens. I value another quality in some of my closest friends: an ability to understand me and identify what I am trying to achieve, to respect that but sometimes to tell me if it is not achievable or if I am going about it the wrong way. I want to be surrounded by people who will tell me what they think, not what they think I want to hear.

My friends know that I have been a full-time carer in recent times. Some approve. A few who have also known me for many years think that I am mad and that I should ensure that Pat is cared for in a different way and return to work. I value all my friends and believe that each of them, regardless of their opinions, shares an equal concern for my welfare. I am glad that those who disagree feel confident enough in the strength of our friendship to express it.

Knowing the personalities of my friends, I am sure that

none of them are saying what they think I want to hear. Many have known Pat as well over the years, so it is more likely that they also know me well enough to know that I feel unable to walk away from this situation and allow someone else to look after Pat.

Some activities are now very difficult. I used to enjoy going to occasional dinners, sometimes more than twenty miles away from home and which finished late. I can no longer do that. In the past I have sat next to people at functions who have had to leave early to look after a younger or older relative. Able at that time to attend and to stay late, I understood their circumstances, but having such responsibility myself is very different. So I am very grateful to those who understand that I am not able to see them as much as I would wish because of my need to put Pat first.

With carers to look after Pat, though, I keep in touch with many people. Most weekdays a carer provides cover for a few hours during the daytime, enabling me to attend to e-mails, make phone calls, go shopping, even write pieces such as this or whatever other activity I might need or want to do.

During the evening I like to relax and spend as much "quality time" as I can with Pat. As I have written in a previous article, both of us enjoy it when I am able to read aloud. Doing so has reminded me that as a child I enjoyed reading animal stories and it has perhaps also introduced me to some interesting books I might not otherwise have read.

Occasionally, "cover" during the evening enables me to meet old friends who are not free during the day. Because of my responsibilities and the consequent need to make arrangements for Pat, such activities are probably even more special to me than they would otherwise be.

One old friend – he might prefer the description "longstanding"! - once told me how abiding he considered true friendship to be: "Your friends are always there." He happens to disagree with the course of action I have taken as regards Pat. Over the years, though, he has been a wonderful (and humbling) example of loyalty.

I want to stay in touch with friends, but at times such contact has to be over the phone or by e-mail rather than face to face. I am grateful that my friends have made every effort to stay in touch with me, too.

I hope that I too can offer advice when needed (and if requested!). A couple, recently retired, were contemplating inviting a close relative, living on their own and now in poor health, to live with them. It is not for me to judge the actions or circumstances of others. However it was only right, given both my experience and our friendship, that I should point out that this might not be an easy course of action. I suggested that they should give careful consideration to the matter, and in particular whether they could cope with a likely deterioration in the health of their relative, before doing so.

I have learned, and continue to learn, from those around me. The most recent period has not been easy, but it would have been considerably more difficult if my life had not been enriched by those I am privileged to call my friends. They both understand and demonstrate the meaning of the word friendship. I have never needed them as much as I do now.

one carers tales no.11

Good Times, Bad Times

...

I would like to think that, in the course of these articles, I have given a balanced picture of my life as a carer. It has been a challenging period. Yet it has also been amusing, at times, and has given me perspectives which I wouldn't otherwise have had.

Over the last five years or so, I have spent more time hospital visiting than in all my other years put together. One parent spent a long time in hospital and then moved to respite but sadly never returned home.

Pat has gone into hospital several times and thankfully the cause has generally been relatively minor complaints. I have perhaps not seen it as such at the time, but it has given me insights into our healthcare system.

Firstly, may I pay tribute to the many wonderful people who work within it? Having many family members who have worked in the NHS over the years this should not surprise me, but I am always struck by how much people seem to care rather than simply doing a job. This is particularly important when sitting in an ambulance, accompanying a sick person to hospital and not knowing what will in due course be diagnosed. I am always struck by the professionalism of ambulance crews. I have no wish to accompany somebody in their vehicles more often than I have to, but I find them very reassuring people.

The care does not stop there, though. It is present in A&E and on the Wards, too. It is present in places of respite, if they are part of the patient's recovery. Its presence lifts some of the burden from the relatives, who can at least be confident that the person they love is being well looked after.

There are, however, aspects of hospital procedure which cause concern, especially when they are looking after older people. I cannot but comment on these, too.

Firstly, patients who will be admitted to a hospital ward spend a lot of time in A&E before they get there. I understand that various tests have to be undertaken, but it would be helpful if explanations were given as to what tests are to be done and the likely timescale. As a relative accompanying an older patient I find this frustrating. How much more so is it for a person who may be confused and have limited understanding of what is happening to them?

Usually I have been at the hospital when discharge has taken place. I am glad I have. If anything, this is even more frustrating. I might spend a couple of hours with Pat, waiting to move to the Discharge Lounge while nobody knows what is happening. There follows an uncertain wait for an ambulance to provide transport, generally to a place of respite for a few days. (Meanwhile I try not to think about the possibility my car might have been parked for a longer period than I have paid for: I defend parking charges if they mean day patients and visitors can get a space, but they can cause problems in some situations).The staff in the Discharge Lounge (as elsewhere in the hospital) are first-class, but they cannot spend all their time looking after one patient. I hate to think of Pat being alone there.

Fortunately Pat has normally left the hospital in the late afternoon. I have seen some elderly patients discharged to their own homes mid-evening, something I have very serious concerns about.

On one occasion, just before discharge, the hospital arranged a meeting with the morning care provider to "assess" Pat's mobility. I found out about this by accident and asked to attend. I was told I could, but the care home into which Pat was to be discharged could not. As it happened, they weren't free to do so: had they wished to attend, I would have supported their request forcefully. No assessment took place: the care provider was shown something in the medical notes, sight of which I was not offered, and proceeded to demand that Pat sleep downstairs in future and have a hoist installed. I believed then that this was wrong: something proved the following day when Pat moved to the care home. It was immediately clear that the lack of mobility had been grossly exaggerated. I still feel sore at the hospital, for failing to check Pat's mobility and organising such a meeting in secret. I am even angrier that the care agency accepted without question what they were told, with no supporting evidence, and sought to lay the law down on that basis. I was tempted to wonder, at that moment, who paid their wages? (I kept the agency: the quality of front-line staff more than compensates for management failings).

I have highlighted failures of management and communication in this piece. Hospitals should have special regard to the needs of older people. They and care agencies should also treat full-time carers as an asset and deal with them on a professional basis.

one carers tales no.12

"Known Unknowns"

...

I am planning a rather different New Year's Resolution, next time I am called upon to make one: to read the Data Protection Act.

A while ago, I contacted a company about an insurance policy, which is in Pat's name, covering pipes etc for which the homeowner is responsible. I quoted the policy number and the somewhat outrageous figure to which the company proposed to increase the monthly premium. I had all the information at my fingertips. Pat finds it difficult to use the telephone and had previously authorised me to speak to and negotiate with this company.

The "operative" at the other end of the line immediately spoke to his manager (why can the customer never speak to the manager?) who apparently reported back that I had dealt with them four years ago. I pointed out that this information was a little incomplete: I assisted them last year to unravel a rather expensive mistake they had made in their own favour and have probably spoken to them about the cost of the policy each year for several years. The operative hastened to point out that he hadn't meant to imply that they had only spoken once to me (which is exactly what it had sounded like): however, they could not negotiate with me about the premiums due to the "Data Protection Act". Pat who, as I have said (and explained patiently to the operative), finds it difficult to use the telephone, needed to give further authority to these people. (My name is on Pat's Bank Account: I could, without reference to this company, cancel the policy as I also pointed out).

On the same day, an hour or so later, I spoke to another insurance company, also regulated by the Financial Conduct Authority (which my friend the operative had also mentioned) on Pat's behalf. Pat had similarly given authority to the second company to speak to me. There, the employee checked their records, asked me a question to confirm my identity and dealt with me. (Admittedly, they didn't give Pat a reduction, but you can't have everything, can you?)

Two different companies, two different interpretations of the Act: surely one of those companies (hopefully the first one) needs to get their lawyers to re-read the Act and understand its purpose?

The most amusing incident with the Data Protection Act, though, was a year or so ago. We ordered an item via a well-known mail order catalogue in Pat's name. They sent the wrong item, together with the name and address of the woman, a complete stranger living thirty miles or so away, to whom they should have sent it.

I telephoned Wellknown Mailorder Co. Plc to make arrangements to return the item to them at no cost to ourselves. I then, not unnaturally, asked when Pat's item would be delivered. I was flabbergasted to be told that they couldn't tell me because of the Data Protection Act. An Act which I felt they had breached in a rather big way as regards somebody else's personal details and, quite possibly, Pat's too. Despite my astonishment, I probably pointed this out when challenging what was being said. On that occasion, I was put through to a manager and given the information.

Not everybody is so hung up about this wonderfully flexible Act. One garage several members of the family dealt with a few years ago (and from which each of us actually bought our cars before having them serviced there) regularly sent the wrong bills to the wrong people in the family. We found it amusing: there might have been circumstances in which it could have been embarrassing.

The Data Protection Act is presumably designed to protect people as well as their data. Perhaps it ought to be called "The People's Data Protection Act", though that name might remind people of fads in the late 1990s rather than their duty to act with common sense in their use of it.

Surely this legislation is not intended to be the modern equivalent of the "Dad's Army" refrain "Don't you know there's a war on?" or its more recent equivalent "I'm afraid I'm having trouble with the computer today".

If I may risk somebody having a fit of the vapours, may we use a little common sense here? (We can put it away soon enough). Surely, the Data Protection Act is not meant to ensure that an insurance company can hide behind it and charge Pat more because, despite having authority to do so, they are unwilling to discuss cutting the premiums with me? Surely they don't seriously think that Pat will take legal advice if they tell me when a delivery is due? All of us know the importance of data protection in modern society. Those who hold our data should concentrate on system security rather than abandoning common sense and embracing a universal modern excuse. One of those still exists anyway: "I'm afraid I'm having trouble with my computer today....."

Update:
The Data Protection Act has now been replaced by the General Data Protection Regulations. Given that a few charities I have supported for many years felt a need to ask for permission even to continue to write to me, I think my request for Common Sense remains a valid one....

one carers tales no.13

Call Centre Workers' Right of Reply

...

I have in previous pieces been very critical of my Bank on occasion. I have referred to the experience of having the words Act, Protection and Data (to quote the right words, but not necessarily in the right order) spoken to me in the most ridiculous circumstances. There was the sadly missed individual who seemed to think that a change of procedure would thwart my effort to get the information I required from one of her colleagues (sadly missed only because she was wrong about that on every occasion....)

These experiences have occurred in the course of dealing with call centres, so the reader may well imagine that I find dealing with companies on the telephone a nightmare (and that, quite possibly though it would be rude to say so, this is reciprocated by those who have to deal with me).

I do find it irritating when I telephone and am greeted by a range of options and button-pushing. The more so when, on occasion, I am using a telephone which doesn't play the button-pushing game and the system does not seem to have a default option for such circumstances: "...or hold the line and you will be put through to the next operator." (The Inland

Revenue didn't merely repeat its options several times a few years ago: it cut me off).

Even more irritating is being asked, say by my Bank, to say in a few words what I want to do: I am then put through a while later to "the next available operator" who doesn't seem to have received this message. At least I presume not: I have never asked. If this is simply a displacement activity while I am waiting to be put through to somebody, as I suspect in some cases the button-pushing is, can we dispense with it?

I don't mind the music, though I find the constant interruption by messages that "your call is important to us" very irritating. Perhaps if they said "your call is nearly important enough for us to employ enough operatives" I would at least respect their honesty!

Don't attempt to sell me anything on the phone while you are wasting my time: "We're sorry you can't get through at the moment: this is probably because millions of people have decided to invest in our brilliant new ISA..." does not endear you, or your product, to me.

The technology seems to exist to tell me whereabouts in the queue I am (or, alternatively, how long I am likely to have to wait): so why isn't it universally used? I have been on the telephone waiting to speak to somebody for half an hour, not knowing whether I am thirty seconds or another thirty minutes away from speaking to customer services.

Please don't tell me that you don't give "advice" when I asked you a factual question.

Most of these deficiencies are those of the management in designing the system (or perhaps in providing insufficient training), not the person I speak to when I eventually get through. I have, occasionally, dealt with difficult people on the phone, more often those who are "management" than the first person I have spoken to on a particular occasion.

The vast majority of calls I have made to Call Centres (including those of my Bank) have been answered by pleasant people who have proceeded to deal with my request in an efficient manner and given me complete satisfaction. This has been true wherever those people have been based. Some have managed more than that: their good humour has left me with a smile on my face, something which the best service can achieve in any situation.

I should add that, in my turn, I try to be as professional in my dealings with them as they are with me. However wretched a company they may be working for – at least as it might seem to me at that moment – that is not the fault of this individual who is (hopefully) trying to help.

The words "Customer Services" have in the past filled me with dread, as I have looked upon it as the department (in whatever organisation) intended to ensure that the one does not get the other. Sometimes, by revealing the limitations of what they can say or do, Call Centre operatives give me the impression that I am right about this.

I probably deal with more Call Centres than I would wish. Many others would probably say the same. What is certainly true is that most people working in them do a good job under pressure. There must be times when they no more enjoy the experience of dealing with us than we do with them.

one carers tales no.14

Raving Bankers...

...

Boris writes: "The Bank has upgraded its software systems", I was told cheerfully this morning by the operative on the other end of the 'phone.

"Downgrade expectations all ye who hear these words", I told myself gloomily.

I wasn't wrong. "My" telephone banker (to whom I am always told I will be put through) proceeded to tell me what the bank couldn't now do which it had always done for me in the past. In this case, it related to putting required references on a transaction I was performing on behalf of Hilary.

I suppose, if the telephone banker belongs to me, so must the Bank. So I should report this is not all "my" Bank has been doing which I should like to let off steam about, whilst making clear that I am not a Grumpy Old Man. Honest.

In common with other Banks, it has been closing Branches and cutting the service at those which remain. So, whereas before in my small town three manned counters served the public five days a week, two now do so every weekday except Wednesdays. This amounts a virtual halving of the service provided: eight-fifteenths of it, if we are going to be pedantic, or if the Bank's Public Relations Officers or Legal Team happen to be reading this.

It is A Truth Universally Acknowledged that everybody should do their banking over the internet says My Bank. "And So Say All of Us", say all of its main high street competitors – and act accordingly.

"I don't believe it", one Meldrew V. would reply if he were a customer. Those waiting in the sometimes long queue to get to the counter are probably in the Meldrew V. School on this one.

Obviously, I would not wish a very busy person to have to wait in the queue. It would be intolerable if the Chief Executive of the Bank, its Chairman or one of its Senior Directors was held up in this way, given their responsibilities and the demands on their time. The Director of Customer Experience, should they have one, would also be a busy person, so let's hope they never have to wait in this way either.

I would like to explain to these important people, though, that there are times when the person at the counter isn't just paying in a cheque or withdrawing some cash or somesuch – here this minute, gone the next. They appear to be telling their life story: or if they aren't, perhaps they should be. It might be quicker than what they are actually doing.

One day earlier this week (it's been that kind of week) a customer in the Branch, was using his mobile phone as well as talking to the cashier. He didn't appear to be multi-tasking – he was a man, after all – as he gave the mobile phone to the cashier, who also spoke to the person at the other end. This might, I am sure, have been entertaining for the dozen or so of us in the queue if we could have heard the conversation – perhaps the phone could have been passed around for us to add our comments? I did catch his address, a breach of his confidentiality no doubt, but who cares about such things these days? As it was, one counter was effectively out of action for a long time and the rest of us moved even more slowly than usual.

Sometimes the Bank stands us in front of the television as a displacement activity, though unfortunately it wasn't switched on that day. It shows twenty-four hour news, sans sound but complete with sub-titles. I entertain myself by looking out for misspellings generated by the computer until it is my turn to move to the counter and get on with my life. You can only distract a childish person like myself for so long with such activity, however.

May I revisit the eighth paragraph of this piece, please? The people standing in the queue at the Bank are its customers. They might be the owners of small businesses on which our local economy depends; grandparents or parents looking after the children for the day; carers like myself, or members of any one of a dozen more categories. They are actually important people – we all are – and no less so than the Chief Executive, Chairman or Director of Customer Experience of the Bank. Our time is no less important or valuable to us than theirs is to any one of those three eminent personages.

We are in the Bank because we either can't do what we want online, don't understand it, don't trust it or don't wish to use it. We have a transaction to undertake. Will the CEO, Chairman or Director of Customer Experience now stop bullying us to use the internet and join the queue – or, even better, do something to mitigate it?

Update:

Lateral thinking can provide for interesting solutions. On a recent visit to my Branch there were at one point fifteen people waiting. I was in the middle of the queue when I counted them and each time somebody left the bank another person seemed to enter it.

I can report that there are no such problems now. Whether I admire the Bank's innovative thinking which has produced this happy state of affairs is a different matter.

They have closed the Branch.

one carers tales no.15

When Larry Met Sybil

...

"I'm Sybil", she purred, sitting down right next to him.

"I'm Lawrence Sebastian", he replied, studying the elegant female beside him.

"How posh".

"Meow", he responded, then added: "Larry for short."

"So what do you do?" she asked.

"Work for the Big Cheese", he replied. "PR work for the Head Honcho. Do you know, when I arrived they wanted me to take responsibility for rodent control as well? How does that fit in with my expertise in Public Relations? 'Rats!' I thought to myself, 'I'm not having that. I prefer to do a little chillaxing in my spare time.' I've got very heavy responsibilities, you know." He was very conscious of them every time he allowed himself to relax near the radiator.

"My boss was the numbers man", she continued. "He provided the money for everything. He worked in the building next door to where you live now. I saw all his secret papers."

"Fell asleep over them, more likely", he sniffed.

"Now who's being catty?" she asked crossly. Not that she denied it....

"We are the Masters now", he replied, trying to change the subject, perhaps a little clumsily. He recalled that somebody important had said something similar back in 1946.

Her boss no longer worked there. Larry had arrived with the New Broom. Sybil didn't entirely like the way things were done now, but now wasn't the time for office politics or philosophy. Larry would no doubt defend his boss – and she did quite fancy him. He was a real Cool Cat.....

Sybil was curious, though, and anxious to change the subject again. Now was not the time for a catfight. "What's he like, your boss?" she asked. "As a person, I mean?"

There we must leave two of the more famous (feline) residents of Downing Street in modern times to our imagination.

This incident, I hasten to add, never happened. It is a product of my imagination. Sybil sadly died about seven years ago. Other (and better) fiction is available.

Worse fiction is available too. (I have probably written some myself). I don't generally expect to receive it through the post, though, in an envelope bearing the logo of a utility company.

The other day I got a pleasant surprise. An unexpected payment had been made into the Bank Account. This apparently related to the gas supply. An overpayment – of an amount larger than two monthly payments – was being returned. Consequently I was not particularly nervous when I opened two letters from the supplier the same day. As some monies had been returned, they couldn't contain bad news, could they?

Both contained the same news. I was pleased to note that the supplier had a grip on their administrative costs. Monthly payments were going up by more than fifty per cent. I rang the supplier, which shall remain nameless. I enquired when they had increased the cost of gas by half. I had understood that energy prices were falling, not rising. I gathered there had been no such increase. Further investigation of my annual statement revealed that, in the company's opinion, I would use about a third more gas over the coming year than I had actually used the previous year. Why, I wasn't entirely sure....

I expected the operative on the other end of the line to have access to the same document. She did not. Her figures showed a slight increase in my likely gas consumption, necessitating a (considerably smaller) rise in monthly payments. These have not long been reduced. The repayment would have almost paid the extra required over the forthcoming period.

Evidently a focus group had decided that repayments should be made if the company holds such an amount to the credit of the customer. I have never sat on a focus group. Given the apparently barmy decisions they sometimes take, perhaps somebody ought to....

So there we are. Fiction can feature in "Carer's Tales" and even letters from utilities. Some might prefer it if it was once again restricted to bookshops (or online, for the benefit of clever people not like me) clearly labelled so we can take it or leave it....

one carers tales no.16

Parking Mad

...

Seven or eight years ago I was startled to hear among the headlines for my local regional television news summary that a major supermarket was to "fine" its customers for a range of parking contraventions. Startled because I understood that it was the role of the state to deal with offences and, where appropriate, hand out fines – not that of private companies.

So startled and distracted was I that – to my intense annoyance – I did not properly hear a piece, before the one referred to, which featured an old friend.

Around six years ago I took a Close Relative of advanced years (let us call that person CR) to see a cousin of similar age living a couple of hours away. CR wanted to break the journey at a motorway service station, part of a national chain, for reasons not involving expenditure of monies. The motorway service station was on a single site accessed via a roundabout and we broke our journey there again upon our return. Whether we also went into the shop and spent any money, I do not recall.

A week later, I received a letter from a company I had never heard of informing me that I had spent five hours and twenty-eight minutes on the premises of Messrs Wellknownmotorwayservicesco and therefore owed them fifty pounds. Momentarily puzzled, I then realised that I must have, by chance, parked in the same parking bay on both occasions. I wrote to them to point this out: given their attempt to extort monies out of me on false pretences, I suggested that they might wish to make a donation of a similar sum to a worthy charity I had heard making an appeal on Radio 4 the previous Sunday. I also requested a letter of apology from the Manager of the service area. (The mind boggles at the thought of how one would spend five hours and twenty-eight minutes at such a place....)

Messrs Parkingextorters wrote back, graciously saying that I didn't owe them the fifty pounds after all, for which I was most grateful, whilst remaining silent as to whether they would be following up my suggestion of a charitable donation. If they did so, I commend their discretion in not boasting about their generosity. The letter from the Manager of the site was clearly lost in the post. I remain uncomfortable that (I presume) they had been able to get my details from a government agency, whether or not (as in this case) on the basis of untruthful information.

Last summer three of us took Pat on holiday and stopped at a service area in North Yorkshire. We were there a little over two hours – not because the place was a hive of massively interesting activity, but because things sometimes take longer with an older person of more limited mobility.

As we left, I noticed a sign saying that the parking time limit was two hours – a time I know we exceeded. Mentally I rehearsed the letter I would be sending to Messrs Parkingextorters Plc, should I have the pleasure of renewing my contact with them after all these years. It would certainly include mention of the considerable sum we had spent on the premises.

I got no such letter. We were parked in the disabled bay and may have been allowed to stay longer there.

Wheelclamping is now, rightly, illegal. The DVLA should not give personal information to private companies. To add insult to injury I understand that they don't even make a profit on it for the taxpayer! The parking extorters cannot, as I understand it, take legal action without the consent of the landowner, so (whether or not that consent is already given in the contract between extorter and operator of the site) the site operator is ultimately responsible for the activities of the extorter. I would like to read the contracts between the supermarkets or motorway services and parking extortion companies. The suggestion that someone has entered into a contract to park for fifty, sixty or seventy pounds, if they park for more than two hours or whatever the stated time might be, is surely a legal fiction to cover the fact that private companies are setting themselves up with quasi-judicial powers to which they are not entitled.

Landowners may now scream that, if people can park with impunity on their land for unlimited periods, customers might not be able to do so. Fair point: why not allow supermarkets, service areas and other such commercial operations to opt in to the local parking warden service, provided that the use of it is clearly indicated on the site and is provided on a commercial basis making a profit for council tax payers? I think that would provide fair and regulated protection for all parties without a government department passing personal data (and quasi-judicial powers) to private companies.

Have I missed something?

Update:

Parking is if anything a "hotter potato" now than when I wrote this piece. I understand that a code of conduct is shortly to be put on a statutory basis so that companies will need to sign up to it in order to obtain personal details from the DVLA.

A retired neighbour recently received a charge notice relating to a car park at a big four supermarket (whose staff in store washed their hands of the matter). Despite being innocent, she paid it to avoid a larger debt. Another friend had a similar experience a while ago. This is wrong and shows the scale of the problem.

HMG won't listen to me but here are some of the provisions a code should contain to be fair to all parties:

- *Ability to pay for parking by cash or card in all cases whether or not more exotic options are available.*
- *A right to park without charge if a machine isn't working unless there are clear directions to a nearby machine which is functioning.*
- *A reasonable period of time (say fifteen minutes?) to obtain a ticket after finding a parking space.*
- *A statutory maximum charge for exceeding the time paid for or other infraction.*
- *A right of appeal to an independent body where a charge notice is issued. The name of the company and contact details (address, phone number and e-mail) should be provided. Victims should be able to contact them easily, receiving prompt response to phone calls or e-mails, to register an appeal. No payment or increase due to delayed payment should*

be due until the outcome of the appeal has been notified.

- *The Big Cheese of a parking organization recently said that the cost of dealing with parking appeals is £25.00. Presumably he considers this a reasonable amount of compensation for victims whose work in defending themselves from wrongly imposed charges is currently unpaid and whose time is equally valuable.*
- *DVLA should be notified where parking companies have obtained details from them on the basis of false information.*
- *If a matter goes to court companies should be required to show evidence that a vehicle was parked throughout the alleged period or of the parking infraction. In 2025 we cannot simply trust technology.*

one carers tales no.17

T' Beeb or not T'Beeb...

...

Many years ago, I toured a local BBC radio station with others. The Government of the Day had had a recent spat with "Auntie" about its coverage of an important issue. The BBC was in the dock and the presenter told us that all who worked for it were now more conscious of how they dealt with such controversies. I said that I supported the BBC, not the Government, trying to sound as if I spoke for sixty million people.

"Olav's a....." (insert supporter of unpopular Opposition) one of my colleagues helpfully told the presenter, who now understood that I spoke for about six people.

Issues, and Governments, come and go. The absence of tension between Government and broadcasters would not be top of the list of qualities I would look for in an ideal society. Governments of all colours do foolish things: they, and Oppositions, should be open to scrutiny.

I have for some years watched "The Apprentice". It is, first and foremost, a game show in which highly intelligent, if colourful, young people are put way outside their comfort zone. Those of us of more modest abilities enjoy their foibles.

A year or so ago teams were collecting specific items, including a skeleton. Seeing a cardboard version in a shop, one of two companions tasked with acquiring this item had a brainwave: didn't that match the description and wouldn't it be a cheaper way of getting it? The other agreed and they carefully checked with a bemused shopkeeper that it was indeed "a full anatomical human skeleton." Sadly, things didn't look quite so simple in the dreaded Boardroom: Lord Sugar pointed out that what they had bought was "not a b... skeleton" and asked one of the purchasers why he had thought it was. "I'm not a Lawyer, Lord Sugar," was the immediate reply, "but my colleague is. I relied on his judgement." A priceless moment on television, and one from which it took me a few minutes to recover my composure.

Less amusing was the successful pressure some years before by the then Conservative Opposition not to allow a new series to be broadcast before the 2010 Election because Lord Sugar, then a Labour Peer, might influence how people voted. (This was before Lady Brady, now a Conservative Peer, was created). The premise was ridiculous: Lord Sugar is hardly cast as Mr Nice-Guy in the programme and in any case let us give the electorate credit for some intelligence. It is not for politicians – Government or Opposition – to tell us what we may watch.

Apparently the present Government doesn't always like the BBC – which is fine by me, as long as that has also been true of all its predecessors, regardless of their political stripe. Whether the BBC schedules "Strictly" or Dr Who against something popular on ITV should not be decided by a Government Minister. Nor should they be able to terminate the Charter at short notice if they dislike something the Corporation does.

Generally I think the BBC seeks to be fair in its political

coverage. Sometimes I am irritated that interviewers do not ask the questions I would like to. Once, Dame Margaret Beckett, in her pre-National Treasure Days, said something so outrageous on "Today" that I would have blamed her if I had had an accident at the roundabout I was navigating in Wakefield; Ed Balls has a question to answer from something he lobbed in at the end of an interview, circa October 2007; Anne Widdecombe first entered my consciousness about twenty-five years ago saying one of the most ridiculous things I have ever heard from a politician. I know: I have no right not to be annoyed....

I don't watch a lot of television, often sitting down to do so for about an hour before assisting Pat to go to bed. I will look for something to interest us both. I have watched many quality BBC programmes – about animals, for example. There was a wonderful documentary a few years ago about a village with fifty three cats, fifty of which had tracker devices fitted and were followed (often on nocturnal sorties into other residents' houses!)

The presenter at the local radio station said all those years ago that political coverage was not the most important thing the BBC did. He was right. Voters don't take instructions from broadcasters either, so mistakes they make (as they do) are unlikely to be catastrophic. Politicians interfere with the BBC at their peril (and ours...)

The BBC, and our ability to watch a range of "freeview" channels, is funded by the Licence Fee. Those who think it shouldn't be should explain, please, how those of the least means would otherwise be able to access such a range of television output for a smaller expenditure.

Update:

As I write this, the BBC is no more popular with the Government of the day than when I wrote the original piece. Broadcasters should aim for the highest standards of integrity. I am not persuaded that abolition of the licence fee will give the poorest in society the range of viewing they have now for the same or lower cost. Unless that case is made, I won't support it.

one carers tales no.18

The Changing of the Guard

...

Boris writes: "Hello. Bigge Carselling Company?"

"I'm sorry, I must have misdialled", I replied, not quite understanding it. "I was ringing the Cuddly Car Company."

"We are the Cuddly Car Company", I was told. There had, apparently, been a takeover a few days earlier. I hadn't noticed anything different that morning, a couple of months or so ago, when I took my car in for a pre-arranged service. Seeing the same friendly face on reception, I had joked that they should be able to find the car within half an hour. I had later rung to request that they let me have the invoice when they returned the car. I like to pay promptly.

Getting a message from Jo the carer a little later that they had rung me, I returned the call. They listed what needed doing (including an item I had specifically asked them to attend to) and said they might need to keep it overnight. They would let me know in an hour or so. A promised further phone call to me was never made and I spent much of the afternoon chasing the garage. It wasn't the best introduction to Bigge Carselling Co., but I was conscious that those at the garage would now be dealing with new procedures and the changeover had been less than a week previously.

A friend reported that another Bigge dealership had not gained the unqualified approval of a colleague but I decided to keep an open mind.

A mind that was perhaps a little less open after a telephone call a month later, suggesting that I might like to have a particular job done within the next few weeks and even – helpfully – telling me precisely when I could take the car in. I pointed out to the person at the other end of the line that my car had been in for a service a month before and nobody had suggested this job needed doing, even though I had spoken to the garage several times during the day. Unconvincingly, he said that it didn't need doing then, but would be a good idea now. Were people at Bigge unaware that car services are generally at yearly intervals now, and most people find it inconvenient to be without their car more frequently than that? I wondered whether my message had got through – or whether he thought it polite to agree with the customer.

I considered whether the work was required and discussed it with friends, whom I trusted and who knew what they were talking about. Despite their unanimous advice to the contrary I decided that not to do the work might be the greater risk. So I booked the car in again.

The day started so well for them. The service receptionist recognised me, although I did not know them, and sorted out the paperwork. I walked off hoping that my view of them might improve. I was out, but Jo the carer had my contact details. I rang her to check that the garage had not been in touch before contacting them about half past three. This was supposed to be a short-ish job.

"Oh, yes, we've done it", replied Bigge. "We rang at ten past twelve."

Not according to Jo, they didn't. I know which one I trust.

So, a little short of time before Jo was due to finish her shift looking after Hilary, I walked to the garage to collect the car. My friend from that morning gestured me to a different receptionist, sitting at a neighbouring desk, who explained the car had been sorted out and handed me the keys.

"Just one thing", said the Bigge man. "We're not allowed to hand over the keys until customers pay." I resisted either pointing out that he just had or making use of what was now in my hand – tempting as both courses of action were.

Slight problem, that. Cuddly never required immediate payment. Unusually, I was not carrying the relevant plastic that day. Something I explained, somewhat apologetically.

"You wouldn't go to Asda and expect to leave without paying for the goods" lobbed in the Leader of the Opposition (no relation to Jeremy Corbyn), sitting diagonally across.

"Il ne faut pas quitter Asda sans payer". I wondered which great French Philosopher was being quoted here? No longer entirely sure which person I was dealing with, I pointed out to my friend (this morning, at least) that Cuddly did not require immediate payment upon collection of the vehicle and that I had in any event planned to pay the bill within the next couple of days.

"We are not Cuddly!" was the reply - an entirely unnecessary comment. Had my literary skills not stretched to reading the signs on the garage which had finally been changed, the failure to return telephone calls, failure to carry out the original service properly and lack of trust of a very long-standing customer would have given me a clue that things had now changed.

A rather exciteable Prime Minister - who was memorably told to his face by an eventual successor that "you were the

Future once" - had the bright idea that those guilty of anti-social behaviour could be marched to cash points to pay their dues to society. Bigge's seemed to have the same idea. I resisted, then gave in – accepting a lift back home to collect the card, return, pay and take my car home – but only after my counter-offer of paying by card over the telephone when I got home had been rejected.

After such a wonderful experience both of pseudo French philosophy and poor customer service, I should be ungrateful indeed if I ceased to deal with a garage whose bills I have been paying for at least twenty-eight years. My parents' dealings went back a further twenty. After all, the distrust between myself and Bigge is clearly mutual. Whilst I might worry that at the next service they might once again forget to do an important job, their directors clearly have sleepless nights wondering if I am going to pay their bill or suddenly disappear to Gretna Green, never to be heard of again.

Yet I now contemplate the unthinkable. There is a good chance I will not use my local garage again. Bigge, in my recent experience, is not Beautifulle....

Update:

I have probably bored many friends to tears with this story, Olav included. Later discovering that part of a wheeltrim was missing, an observant neighbour told me that it had disappeared around three months before – about the time of the service – and it could only have happened when a wheel was removed from the car. Bigge had changed a tyre.

A different garage serviced my car the following year. A while later Bigge promoted somebody who had impressed me in Cuddly days to be head of servicing at their garage. I decided that – rather than continuing to dine out on this amusing story – I would see whether they were willing to put matters right. In company of a friend, who was still a Bigge customer, I made an appointment. The (now) Bigge man said all the right things to us and I looked forward to receiving a positive message from him in due course.

There was no e-mail or phone call. I chased him for a response. My guess is he wanted to do the right thing but was stopped by management from doing so.

I have since changed my car. I did not even consider the local dealer.

one carers tales no.19

Money Money Money...

...

I assist Pat with Financial Management in the broadest sense. Thus, for example, I may ring up the provider of some type of household insurance if the annual renewal has been pitched at an unreasonable level, as it often seems to be. I organise the hours for Gerda, the carer, and ensure there are sufficient funds in the relevant bank account to pay her. Some of my experiences in dealing with these matters have featured in previous "Carer's Tales".

Gerda is directly employed by Pat and – with the help of a payroll company – I deal with the administration. Most readers will be aware that recent changes in legislation oblige employers either to offer a pension or to provide one, depending on the income of the employee.

I once thought – but probably didn't express the opinion aloud – that if ever I started to listen to Radio Four's "Moneybox", friends should arrange for me to be put out of my misery as soon as possible. I will therefore gloss over the identity of a radio programme which I now regularly listen to around Midday on a Saturday.....

I was listening to that unnamed programme, while travelling

some distance to see an elderly relative, when I received my first information about the new pension regulations. I was grateful for this as I had been aware of the changes in the law but was unsure how they would affect Pat and Gerda. After listening to the programme I had a very clear idea.

Gerda, I gathered, was earning insufficient to be covered by the requirement to pay into a pension scheme and to receive employer's contributions. I subsequently gathered that HM Revenue and Customs had sent some information – to the "payroll people" rather than to Pat. They evidently took the view that, since the payroll people deal with the paperwork around payments to Gerda, they would deal with the pension aspect also. I was surprised at this assumption: the fact that the company provides one (practical) function does not necessarily mean that clients wish to take (and pay for) advice from them on other matters.

The question of employer pensions had been one that had concerned me for some time before that. Being that I am not a large multi-national company with a more than adequate legal/accountancy function – or indeed a medium-sized enterprise – I would have preferred it if HMRC had sent the information somewhat earlier to Pat, so that decisions could be made as to whether additional expert advice and guidance was required or not.

On a separate matter, I took out my own private pension with a "Blue Chip" provider some time ago, when my circumstances were a little healthier and I was able to make contributions to it. A couple of years ago I was approached by a representative of said company, requesting that he visit, review my circumstances and provide any appropriate advice arising out his call. Having taken relevant details, he advised me to switch to a different product within his company's portfolio, as management charges would be less and therefore there should be a greater return.

I asked what I considered to be a very relevant question - would the new pension have the same investment managers? He replied that it would not, but that this made no difference. I am not a financial expert, but I was not entirely convinced. The return, it seemed to me, was very heavily dependent on the investment managers, and I was being asked to gamble that new ones would perform as well as those on the previous policy. Fees for the advice would be taken from – and therefore deplete – the pension fund. I was not able to make new contributions to that pension policy – even to the limited extent of the amount payable for the advice – and so felt particularly vulnerable.

Nevertheless, my lack of financial expertise meant that I followed the professional advice – and I will, of course, never know whether I would have been better off not doing so.

I can only conclude that, for most of us, some financial transactions are very easy, but some are not. We all have to make our own decisions regarding our pensions and hope that we make good decisions. Gerda, in fact, had the option – but was not required – to take a workplace pension.

It would be helpful, though, if the cared for – or indeed those who help them look after their monies – were assisted by the authorities now that they find themselves in the position of being employers, without the resources generally available to the latter.

one carers tales no.20

An Electric Shock & Do I Make Myself Clear?

...

A while ago an unexpected (and considerable) credit in Pat's bank account was, I discovered, a repayment from the electricity company. Two bits of good news rolled into one, for this windfall surely meant that there would be no nasty shocks when the bill arrived?

If only life were so simple! The bill, received shortly afterwards, announced prominently on its first page that the monthly direct debits would be increasing substantially. The electricity supplier, had simultaneously made a refund and increased monthly payments (but without keeping its costs under control by advising of these two moves under the same cover). I was shocked by this and wondered if this bizarre combination was the consequence of a mistake on the part of the supplier. I rang up to check on the situation and was assured that everything, including the increase, was correct.

Let me just restate what the electricity company had done, varying the wording slightly. Over the course of twelve months, Pat had paid by direct debit for more electricity than had been used. The company, having held on to that surplus for up to twelve months (and any interest earned on it) then refunded it at the end of the accounting period, rather than using it to pay for further units of electricity to be credited to Pat's account against future use. Having repaid the surplus, it proceeded to charge for those units of electricity, previously paid for by Pat but unused, at a higher price. (Please correct me if anything in this description of Powerco's activities is factually inaccurate).

I am not sure whether this action on the part of the company is caused by a focus group (of which there was some suggestion) or government legislation. What I do know is that this is very unfair.

Any overpayment by a consumer to a utility company should be dealt with by an option to use that as a credit against units of electricity or gas at the price current when the payment was made. I am quite happy for customers to have a choice of a refund if they so wish.

*

Corporate communications and actions as well as their terms of business should be clear accurate and easily understood by ordinary people. So should signs and notices aimed at the general public. I leave readers to judge whether the following are good examples of the application of those principles....

During lockdown I started to use a small Post Office locally instead of the large one in the town. It felt safer at that time and, although well used, was generally also much quicker. A while later a notice from the Post Office announced the postmaster had resigned and suggested people use the large post office "during this period." Did this mean closure was temporary, as those three words implied, or permanent? I hoped the ambiguous words meant the former but suspected and feared the latter (as proved to be the case). Why didn't the PO just state in their notice that it had closed down?

I can't buy a railway ticket online without ticking a box to confirm I have read the terms and conditions of the train operator. So am I asked if I have read the t&cs when, more usually, I buy tickets at a ticket office? Never. Perhaps the two classes of railway passengers are not as we imagine them to be....

I guess the terms, which will have been drafted by clever lawyers, state how long a ticket is valid for (as shown on the face of it), what is promised and what definitely isn't (a seat) and provide for what happens if things go spectacularly wrong. They may, of course, be more exciting than my usual bedtime reading (or they may equally be an excellent cure for insomnia). Lest this be taken as an admission that I, unlike other passengers, may have perjured myself – no comment – my address is 10 Downing Street SW1 if anyone in authority wishes to discuss the matter with me. To prove that I am not making this address up, I have a cat called Larry. Honest...

A few years ago a Professor (I think) travelled from Durham to London by train but got off at Darlington, where the fun started, on his way back. He was told that, because his return ticket was to Durham and he had got off early, somewhat bizarrely he had incurred a surcharge, which he refused to pay. Court proceedings were ultimately issued though I believe matters were later settled between the parties. Which I was sorry to hear. I wanted a judge to throw out the case against the good Professor, hopefully accompanied by thunderous words directed at the train company for such a term which defies all logic.

A while ago in a familiar place which will remain nameless we looked at a market we hadn't seen before. Why I'm not sure – I suspect it wasn't my idea. A long list of regulations outside the building made it clear that desisting from a specified anti-social activity if so requested by a Police officer was an offence. I reread it several times and a companion confirmed I had read it correctly. While I suspect it doesn't give legal protection to those engaging in whatever the exciting activity was – sadly I can't remember - I hope this brilliantly drafted sign has the equivalent of listed building status. I would hate to see it removed….

one carers tales no.21

On Money and Matters Medical...

...

I mentioned in the introduction that one of my parents died as the other was becoming frail, both physically and mentally. This meant that, almost without notice I was plunged into managing Pat's affairs. A while later twenty-four hour care would become necessary.

I needed to get to grips urgently with Pat's finances and ensure that I could make necessary payments – something else to do at a difficult time – but I knew from our earlier dealings that Pat wanted me to do so should such circumstances arise. Now they had. If Pat thought I could do it....I was sure I could.

Much of the task was practical. I put as many of Pat's bills as possible on direct debit, which involved a few phone calls (and a lot of patience!) once the bank account was in joint names. Beyond this, I made few changes, though there remained quite a few cheques to write, cheques to pay into the bank and cash to be withdrawn at times. There were, of course, new transactions to set up involving the various carers who would support me in looking after Pat.

Pat had always been generous, enjoying the conversation

and giving, for instance, when current undergraduates rang a member of their University's Class of Many Years Before. Now there were carers to be paid and finances would be much tighter. When I was used to (literally) minding someone else's business and felt that matters were under control, it seemed right to support a few causes close to Pat's heart. So I created some standing orders, spread out over the year, in favour of the University and a small number of charities. I gained great pleasure from this. The gifts were not large but I believe Pat (who would not have used standing orders to do this) would have approved of being able to continue to give.

Running Pat's finances was challenging at times – I have described some of the frustrations in other pieces – but I never lost sleep over any of the decisions I took. Pat might have done things differently, but all bills were paid and any discretion I had I used to try to reflect what Pat would have wanted me to do.

There was another aspect of care for which, I must confess, I feel much less qualified: expressing opinions on matters medical. This was first to put to the test a long time ago.

One of my parents faced an operation previously described to patient and visitors alike at the bedside as "high risk." I don't necessarily need that term to be further defined. The consultant (in whose medical abilities I did not doubt) chose to summon me from work to the bedside to elaborate further. It was more information than I would have wanted, but I was more concerned for the two other listeners, the patient and another visitor. Not getting an immediate reaction, the Consultant said: "Let's see what Olav thinks...."

"Let's not!" jumped in the patient immediately. "I don't want to burden him with it!" An interesting reaction as the patient's hearing was not always good at that time.

The patient consented. I spoke to the Consultant privately afterwards. At my request he set out the alternative to the operation. "You asked what I thought," I told him. "You've made the case. I support it."

On a number of occasions when Pat was in hospital, doctors set out various hypothetical situations in which they would not want to treat Pat further. The case they made was not unreasonable. If the situation had arisen, I would not have criticised their (in)actions.

I am sure that Pat, who managed finances well when in good health and could easily have managed mine if needed, would also have been able to deal with such requests for consent dispassionately if I had been the patient. For me, the comment made many years ago was right, though: I am happy to be burdened with somebody else's finances. Life and death is another matter….

one carers tales no.22

Getting A(nother) Life

...

My work has, at times, given me an insight into the interesting lives of people I haven't met.

There are also aspects of the lives of our nearest and dearest of which we may be unaware. My parents used to receive a lot of Christmas cards. During Pat's first Christmas alone, I had the job of responding (and advising of the year's sad news). Some who had sent cards were familiar faces; some, names I had heard in conversation; some, people I hadn't even heard of. The bad news that year was that Marie, and a couple called Philip and Marie, didn't get cards, because I couldn't work out who they were. (People, not unnaturally, don't usually write surnames on cards to close friends. Less helpful if somebody else has to reply of course…). The good news, that everybody else who sent a Christmas card to my parents also received one that year.

Over the years, I have continued to send Christmas cards to Pat's friends who have stayed in touch – a dwindling bunch, I am sad to report, and in most cases I don't know the story of those who are no longer in contact. I have telephoned a few of those I didn't know to find out their stories and their connections to my parents.

Christmas cards are not the only insight into the lives of my parents. When one of my parents died, a considerable amount of mail addressed to them continued to arrive for quite a long time. Much of it was from charities which, however worthy, could no longer be supported. Where possible, I contacted them to let them know. Some of it was junk mail which needed to be stopped.

A lot of charities were writing to Pat too (whose post I was now also dealing with), along with businesses whose goods and services were no longer relevant. There were too many charities to support in the changed circumstances, but a few caught my eye, including one I had never heard of: Book Aid International.

For several years, I had helped with a Christmas Tree Appeal, an effort by a local voluntary group to collect presents for children who would otherwise be unlikely to receive them. Pat had always given generously to this – books considered to be educational and worth reading. So recent years had reminded me, if I was ever tempted to forget, the value my surviving parent placed on literacy. It seemed an appropriate charity to continue to support and was one of those (as mentioned in the previous piece) in whose favour I set up a standing order. I now give to it too.

At times I have met people locally who have asked me to pass on their regards to Pat. It is easy enough to be polite and pretend we know people's names when we don't. "Just remind me….," I had an excuse to say, and always did under those circumstances – even when, as was often the case, I had never met them before. Perhaps I ought to do that even if they don't want me to pass on their regards to others…..

Old letters and photographs also give fascinating insights

into the lives of our parents.

"Who Do You Think You Are?" asks a well-known television programme and answers it for usually well-known faces.

Discovering more about our parents' lives – people with whom we have shared so much time yet who are part of a different generation – can be fascinating and I have certainly appreciated the opportunity.

Having shared some experiences of my life as a carer, I would now like to share a few memories of more carefree times.

I have called these "Family Treasures". I hope you enjoy them.

one carers tales no.23

Family Treasures I

...

While staying the week with my Aunt Danni – Dad's Sister – in London, we ventured one evening to a different part of London to see my Cousin Patricia, Mum's niece.

Dad took the job of parking his car seriously. I never saw him get out a tape measure to see how far it was from each corner of a space, but he certainly liked to line up his vehicle. While he was doing so, Mum and Aunt Danni got out of the car and rang the doorbell. I kept him company.

The rest of the party were relaxing in Patricia's sitting room by the time Dad and I joined them. We had often met colleagues or friends of Cousin Patricia when visiting her on these occasions so I was not surprised that there was a lady there I didn't know. Unfortunately we had missed the introductions.

I remember little of the conversation from that evening more than forty years ago. I do recall that Patricia mentioned the 1950s criminal case of *R. v Craig and Bentley*, controversial at the time I understand (and shocking to hear about a quarter of a century later). Its outcome is completely discredited now.

It is my memory of a different conversation which I consider to be a family treasure.

In the middle of dinner, Mum turned to the “stranger” (who was, it has to be said, very good company) and told her: “I used to manoeuvre your Father out of bed.” This remark would be something of a conversation stopper at the best of times, I suspect: for anyone knowing my Mother, the impact would be considerably more startling.

This was the first time in the course of the evening I was aware that Mum had met the lady before. There was, I then realised, only one person the stranger could be: my Cousin Barbara, of whom I had heard but had never met, daughter of my Mother’s late Brother Jack.

Conversation moved on to other topics, as it does. At the end of the evening my parents, Aunt Danni and I returned to the car to return to Aunt Danni’s.

As we were setting off, my Father asked: “Who was the lady staying with Patricia?”

Mum explained. It was indeed my Cousin Barbara. I was amused at the thought that my Father (who would have met my Cousin at least once before, at my parents’ wedding) had not worked this out from my Mother’s comment.

“Who did you think it was?” I asked.

“I didn’t know,” he replied sheepishly.

Pure comedy gold....

I recall another comic incident involving my Father, a year or so earlier. I was doing a German Exchange, and we were spending a week in Scarborough during the stay of my German penfriend Conrad. My parents had a copy of a German translation of an Agatha Christie, possibly “The Man in the Brown Suit”, which Dad suggested to Conrad he might read to us in the hotel lounge. Conrad began to do so – and Dad began to drift off to sleep (and to snore, I suspect....)

I'm not sure how much benefit I - or indeed my Mother, who had studied German at night school - got from *"Der Mann im braunen Anzug"*. I suspect that both of us were aware that the person who had asked Conrad to read was most certainly not benefitting from it. Neither of us liked to suggest to Conrad that he bring proceedings to a halt – and he continued completely unfazed. How the exercise was brought to a close I don't now remember….

My Father did a demanding job and his sleep was interrupted at times. He probably had a good excuse for falling asleep on that occasion but it certainly made for a most amusing memory!

one carers tales no.24

Family Treasures II

...

My Mother talked a lot about Germans – three in particular.

Living in a town which suffered much during the Second World War, Mum and her family were bombed out of their home – a story I heard a few times as a child and a situation which I find hard to imagine. What was perhaps most interesting was the way in which the story was told – that Hitler had bombed the house, as if Fuehrer had been flying the plane himself on that occasion. So told, it seemed to take responsibility away from those who had carried out the action and attach the blame to their Leader.

At School I specialised in Languages, studying German at O' Level and later to A' Level. To say that I wasn't dissuaded from doing this by my parents, who lived through that sad conflict, is an understatement. Somebody else in the household had already blazed a trail. My Mother learned German at evening class many years before I began to study it. Several times while I was at Primary School my parents toured with a caravan in various European countries including Germany. We were met by nothing but kindness by locals, in an era where a tragic past would have been in the living memory of many.

Shortly after I started at Secondary School my parents decided to go along the Romantische Strasse in Germany, staying initially in the medieval walled town of Rothenburg ob der Tauber. We then moved on to Fussen, from where we visited the "fairy tale castle" of Neuschwanstein. Those who have seen the 1960s film "Chitty Chitty Bang Bang" will have seen both those locations, fused together to create a single background though they are about seventy miles apart.

On our way down the rather steep hill from the castle, we were in single file: I was sandwiched between my Father at the front and my Mother at the back. Dad and I were blissfully unaware that Mum had fallen – until "a couple of hefty Germans" (as Mum loved to call them) had helped her up, raised their hats, said "Guten Morgen" and hurried on their way, passing us.

Mum told this story much more frequently than that of events thirty years or so earlier.

As mentioned in the previous piece we stayed for a week in Scarborough a few years later with my German penfriend Conrad and my Aunt Danni. The latter volunteered to go for an early morning walk with my very energetic visitor. She arrived in the foyer of the hotel after he did, to be greeted with a glance at his watch and the words: "You are five minutes late!"

This story was relayed to my parents, probably in private, during the course of the day. Mum did not intend to have the same greeting. She arrived five minutes earlier than the agreed time, earlier than Conrad who duly apologised for being late.

I was always impressed by Mum's lack of bitterness that her family had lost their home in that conflict. I was encouraged to have a positive attitude towards Germany and – since I chose to specialise in Languages – to do a German exchange.

My German penfriend's parents and their generation had of course lived through that conflict too. While I was there, they didn't always adhere to a very strict instruction my parents had given me (and which I kept): "Don't Mention the War." I'm glad the older Germans chose to talk about it. It was clear that it had been an unhappy and dangerous experience for them. Most poignant of all was walking through a wartime cemetery with a German Mother who said: "Warum?" – Why?

I grew up in a very different world from that of my parents and their generation. Younger people reading this will shake their heads in astonishment at the world I am recalling through the eyes of an older generation. I am glad that my parents showed by their example that wounds are there to be healed. It is one of many valuable things they taught me.

one carers tales no.25

Family Treasures III
Mind Your Language

...

My Father went round the table asking us what we wanted to eat.

"Fish and chips....?"

He turned to the waiter: *"Poisson et pommes de terre frites s'il vous plait."*

After a few minutes the waiter looked at him quizzically: "Excuse me, Sir, are you English?"

My Father confirmed that he was.

"Well, why the ....are you speaking French then?"

A reasonable question. I am not a regular at the *Pomme d'Or* in St Helier Jersey (which, I discovered many years later, has an interesting part in the island's history). That occasion – during my summer holidays before going to secondary school – was my only visit there.

The words of the waiter may incidentally have been slightly more nuanced. I remember the incident, but not the precise words used, and that was how my Father always told the story afterwards.

We were staying in Dinard in Brittany, from where we had booked a local excursion visiting Jersey for the day. The party, all other members of whom were French, had been dropped off at the hotel in the middle of the day to get some lunch. Golden apples were not on the menu, though I suspect that if lunch wasn't included in the price of the excursion diners would have had to cross the palms of the proprietors of that fine hotel with a considerable amount of silver.

My Father loved languages, as I do, and he also loved Italy and its people. In later years he often went there with my Mother.

I wish I'd been there when he ordered *"Café con Letto."* Readers have no reason to know – I didn't when I first heard the story – that this translates as "Coffee and a bed." What he meant was *"Café con Late"*, white coffee.

Understandably the waiter would have been somewhat taken aback by such a request, in the middle of the day, from a retired couple. Interestingly my Mother, who unlike him had not spent several years attending Italian evening classes, understood what he had said.

As told, the waiter gave my Father "an old-fashioned look." I would like to have seen it.

A well loved local Italian restaurant was for us a venue for special family occasions – birthdays or Christmas time. It was an opportunity for my Father to practise his knowledge of the language on a real live Italian (as his teacher was but other classmates of course weren't). He would do so with relish and the proprietor enjoyed the conversation.

However, such was his enthusiasm he would sometimes say something to a waitress who would point out to him that she didn't understand a word of the language.

One language none of us ever studied was Dutch. Aged twelve I recall arriving in Rotterdam on the way back from a trip to Bavaria. We were due to stay at a motel near the airport before catching a ferry back the following day.

It was well known that Dutch people speak good English so my Mother didn't expect a problem when she asked the petrol attendant how to get to the airport. In English. A language he didn't speak. Second attempt, French. No joy. Third try, German, which she had studied for some time at evening class and a language which it was assumed was vaguely similar to Dutch. Didn't work.

Running up and down the forecourt flapping arms to look like an aeroplane apparently did though quite how the instructions to get there were then communicated I can't quite remember.

Yet another memory which proved to be a family treasure though.

Printed and bound by CPI Group (UK) Ltd, Croydon, CR0 4YY
12/12/2025
02018311-0001